How I Reversed My Hashimoto's Thyroiditis Hypothyroidism

How I Reversed My Hashimoto's Thyroiditis Hypothyroidism

Compiled by Robert T. Dirgo
and
edited by Mary Dirgo

Writers Club Press
San Jose New York Lincoln Shanghai

Writers Club Press
an imprint of iUniverse.com, Inc.

For information address:
iUniverse.com, Inc.
5220 S 16th, Ste. 200
Lincoln, NE 68512
www.iuniverse.com

ISBN: 0-595-16708-X

DEDICATION

I dedicate this book to my dearly beloved wife, Mary Beth. Her constant love and support have enabled me to successfully improve my Thyroid condition as well as make it possible to share my story in this book. God truly opened the heavens and poured out his blessings upon me when he brought her into my life.

CONTENTS

ACKNOWLEDGEMENTS

I want to acknowledge the physician who played a significant role in the reversal of my Thyroid Disease. Dr. Jeffrey Starre is a rare gem of a physician, who is open to alternative methods of attacking traditional problems. I don't know where I would be today if not for Dr. Starre.

I would also like to give a special thanks to Mary Dirgo, President of Galilee Enterprises for her diligent efforts in painstakingly editing this manuscript.

INTRODUCTION

This book is akin to a road map describing my journey from being diagnosed with Hashimoto's thyroiditis Hypothyroidism, to being completely free of thyroid antibodies. I think it would be an interesting read for anyone diagnosed with Hashimoto's who is open-minded enough to consider alternative methods of treatment. Sufferers of non-autoimmune originated Hypothyroidism, may also enjoy reading about some alternative benefits to the thyroid gland.

If you are someone who believes that nothing is impossible, and when you are told that it can't be done, you hear instead, this is going to be an interesting challenge, then this book is for you.

When I was first diagnosed with Hashimoto's and I began my investigation into the disease, I was disappointed to find such despair in my fellow Hashi' sufferers. I recall posting a question on a web page, dedicated to thyroid issues, about solutions for eliminating the source of the problem. Namely, eliminating whatever set off the immune system to attack itself. To me this seemed pretty straightforward. However, I was surprised to see the level of despair that existed. I received unanimous responses basically saying that it's hopeless. There is nothing that can be done. You will just continue to get worse and worse until you have absolutely no function at all in your thyroid.

That just didn't make sense to me! So I set out to find a way to improve my own condition and in turn my quality of life. From a scientific standpoint, it seemed obvious that to properly battle this disease, I would want to focus on the root cause of the problem, not the symptoms. All I heard from everybody I questioned was a focus on the symptoms.

I will outline for you what worked for me. I make no claim that what I did will work for you or any sufferer of Hashimoto's. It may or it may not. If, after reading this book, you don't think you've found a solution to your disease, then at least be encouraged that possibilities exist for reversing Hashimoto's. Your solution may be something different. Never give up or stop trying. God has great plans for us all. Remember, with God all things are possible.

Finally, I would like to devote this book to my lovely and gracious wife Mary Beth. She was with me throughout my diagnosis and journey to recovery. I couldn't have done it without her!

WHAT IS THE THYROID?

I am not a Doctor and I was clueless about the Thyroid Gland when I was diagnosed with Hashimoto's. I just hate it when I don't understand something that affects my daily life, especially when it affects my health. Therefore for the past three years I have done almost non-stop research into finding out what the Thyroid Gland is, how it affects the body, and what happens when disease sets in. What I intend to share with you in this chapter is what I have learned from my research. It is coming to you from the perspective of a layman who is a sufferer of Hashimoto's. Please do not consider this information a substitute for a medical professional. I did not. It is of the utmost importance in your treatment of Hypothyroidism that you obtain a doctor who respects you and that you can trust. To maximize your probability of success, you can help your doctor by becoming as knowledgeable about the thyroid and Hypothyroidism as possible. That is where this book can be of some benefit to you. In addition to sharing my story with you, I will provide you with a plethora of sources for additional Thyroid orientated information to start you on your research journey. You will have no excuse for being misinformed about the thyroid.

The Thyroid Gland

I was astounded to find out how important the Thyroid was to the functioning of the body. I wondered why it was not more well known and respected. The population in general has a great appreciation for the Heart, the Liver or Kidney, all critical organs in the body. Even the Pituitary and the Adrenal Glands have a minimal amount of name recognition amongst the public, although most would not know what they did. But the Thyroid Gland? Who even cares about the Thyroid Gland? I don't think anybody really gives credence to the Thyroid Gland until stricken with a disease. I am here to tell you that the Thyroid "rates" when it comes to importance to the body. In fact, the body could not function without it.

The Thyroid itself is a small butterfly shaped gland located in the lower neck near the Adams apple. (Reference Figure 1) The function of the thyroid is to absorb iodine, which got into the bloodstream from foods containing it. The process, which then takes place within the thyroid, is an interaction between the absorbed iodine and the amino acid L-Tyrosine. This interaction produces the thyroid hormones T4 and T3, which the thyroid gland disperses back into the blood stream. These hormones affect every living cell in the body and they regulate our metabolism. If our metabolism shuts down so do we. You cannot get much more important than that. Perhaps the reason that the Thyroid has not received top billing in years past is that people typically did not have as many problems as currently being experienced. Alternatively, symptoms were misdiagnosed and attributed to other diseases. Nevertheless, it seems that more and more of us are being challenged with Thyroid problems requiring an increased vigilance.

Pituitary Gland

The Pituitary Gland works in concert with the Thyroid Gland. An appropriate analogy would be to consider the Pituitary Gland to be serving the same role as the thermostat does in a heating system. Further, consider the T3 and T4 hormones as being the heat and the Thyroid Gland as the furnace pumping out the heat.

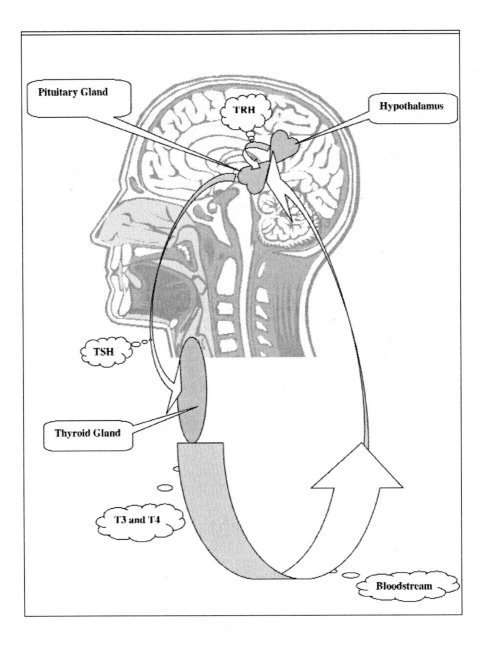

Figure 1

Completing the analogy, our bloodstream would be akin to the room in the house, which has the thermostat. Therefore, when the thermostat of the body, the Pituitary Gland, detects that the bloodstream is low on heat or T3 and T4, then it kicks in the Thyroid Gland to produce more T3 and T4 and pump it into the bloodstream. When the Pituitary Gland determines that enough hormones have been put into the bloodstream, it kicks the Thyroid back off, stopping the flow of thyroid hormones.

In our analogy the thermocouple, which kicks off the Thyroid Gland, is a hormone called TSH. Where TSH stands for Thyroid Stimulating Hormone. The Pituitary gland produces this hormone which motivates the Thyroid to crank out the thyroid hormone.

Hypothalamus

The hypothalamus is the part of the brain that tells the Pituitary Gland to stimulate the Thyroid Gland. It does this with it's own hormone called TRH. Where TRH stands for TSH Releasing Hormone. This part of our analogy can be thought of as the temperature setting.

If the Hypothalamus, Pituitary Gland and the Thyroid Gland are all functioning properly the body just keeps churning along. When the heating system fails, whether it is the thermostat, the furnace or the thermocouple, you do not have heat.

What this book is going to primarily focus on is problems with the Furnace, or the Thyroid Gland. In particular what happens when the furnace slows and does not pump out enough heat. This is known as Hypothyroidism. There are various types of Hypothyroidism. The one that I was diagnosed with is Hashimoto's Thyroiditis.

Hashimoto's Thyroiditis

Hashimoto's is named after the doctor who discovered it, Hakaru Hashimoto. With Hashimoto's the cause of the furnace slowing is attributed to a malfunction of the body's immune system. The body's natural defenders, antibodies, start attacking the thyroid because they misidentify body tissue for that of a foreign invader. In Hashimoto's the target of the antibodies is the Thyroid Gland. The relentless attack of the antibodies wears down the Thyroid such that it becomes less productive in regards to thyroid hormone. This is what is commonly referred to as an under-active Thyroid.

There are other diseases of the Thyroid, which can totally disrupt the homeostasis of the body. Hyperthyroidism occurs when the Thyroid Gland becomes overactive, cranking out too much Thyroid Hormone. There are other variations of Thyroiditis as well, however I am not as familiar with them. The focus of this book is on Hashimoto's Thyroiditis, because that was what I was diagnosed with. I hope you enjoy the ride as you join me on my journey from my descent to disease followed by my rise to recovery.

Just Remember that you are not alone in the world with this disease. Millions have gone before and are out there experiencing the same struggles you do. Some of the more famous individuals that have been stricken with this disease are, President George Bush and First Lady Barbara Bush, Rod Stewart, Tipper Gore, Gail Devers, Faith Ford, Muhammed Ali, Carl Lewis, Ben Crenshaw, Pat Bradley, Patty Berg and Joe Piscopo. These people have shown us all that you can live a very fulfilling life while suffering from Thyroid disease. Keep the Faith!

The Spiral Down to Disease

I never thought of myself as being unhealthy. It just sort of crept up on me gradually and quietly. At a relatively young age I became sensitive to the state of my health and the importance of expending the necessary energy to maintain it at a high level. My father's health was the primary factor in this state of mind. You see my father had his first heart attack at the age of 50. That means that I was fourteen. My father was always active and had a traditional American diet of meat and potatoes and other "good" things. However when he had a heart attack at the young age of fifty, some behavior changes were implemented in our household. He quit smoking the cigars and chewing tobacco and cut back from two beers at dinner to one. Our family also began to watch what we ate a little closer. This was the beginning of a lifelong education on the effect of different foods on cholesterol, fat, blood pressure and other cardiac related aspects of the body. These awareness-raising efforts were accelerated significantly when my father had his second heart attack two months later. Whoa Nelly! This required some serious consideration as to what was causing these attacks and what can be done to prevent them.

Amazingly, some twenty-seven years ago, when treating cardiac problems with diet was hardly heard of, my father decided to do that very thing. In fact, he was encouraged by doctors to have by-pass surgery while he was still young enough, so that it wouldn't be such a trauma on his body. This was at the time when open-heart surgery was being touted as a significant breakthrough in the treatment of heart disease. With all the pressures of accepting this recommendation for surgery, a young father of four, my father, courageously chose to take a different path. That path was to treat his heart condition with diet and exercise. Now twenty-seven years later, my father is in great health and lives a very fulfilling life, enjoying his grandchildren.

This is not to say that those with heart conditions, who are advised to have open-heart surgery, should ignore the recommendations of their doctor. Rather, it only accentuates the point that there is more than one way to skin a cat. My father pursued his regimen of diet and exercise under the direction of his physician, who respected his decision to not have the invasive open-heart surgery.

Our family diet changed significantly. We became extremely concerned with eating foods that were low in fat and/or cholesterol. This meant no eggs, cheese, whole milk, bacon, little red meat and any other fat producing foods. I felt extremely fortunate in a weird sort of way that I was benefiting from this healthy diet at such a young age. I thought that I was going to be ahead of the game, health-wise, from the average person as a result. For years that seemed to be the case. All of my checkups indicated that my cholesterol level was low, at one point, approximately 125, and I always had healthy blood pressure.

I was bound and determined not to have the same health problems my Dad experienced. Therefore in addition to the diet modifications, I incorporated a regimen of exercise into my daily routine. I wanted to do as much aerobic exercise as possible in order to keep those blood vessels flowing with cool clear plasma. I started riding my bike around the neighborhood and then longer distances. I thought, the longer the better. I would go for twenty or thirty mile bicycle trips without even blinking an eye. Later in life when I was in college, I decided to ride my bike back and forth to school. The only thing is that my school was twenty-six miles away.

This pre-occupation with aerobic exercising branched out into running. I became a part of the running revolution, which was, and for that matter, still is, exploding in our country. I started small by running around the neighborhood for a couple of miles. I came to find out that I really enjoyed this running thing and steadily increased my distance. The euphoria I felt from running was unexplainable and I eventually came to associate it with what is referred to as the runner's high. I never was a very fast runner, but I liked to go for the distance. I eventually decided to enter a road race. The first race I entered was a half-marathon. It was called the Peace Race, and it was held in Youngstown, Ohio. I did not break any records or win any medals, but I did finish! That was like winning the gold medal at the Olympics for me!

My love for running continued to blossom and I entered numerous other races. Mostly five or ten kilometer races. I came to the point though, where I wanted to try the granddaddy of all road races. I wanted to run a marathon! So I signed up to run the God's Country Marathon in Coutersport, Pennsylvania. Again I did not break any records, but this time I did receive a medal for finishing seventh in my age division! This honor to me was not diminished by the fact that there were only seven people in my age division that even finished the race!

I continued with my aerobic exercise regimen, eventually incorporating biking, running and swimming into the challenging event of the triathlon. This event consisted of swimming (1) kilometer, biking (40) kilometers and then running a ten-kilometer race. I finished this race, but with no medal. I eventually went on to complete four marathons thus far, one triathlon and numerous five and ten kilometer runs.

On the surface, I thought that this discipline of aerobic exercise, which I incorporated into my life, was kind of like an insurance policy for good health! I came to find out differently, as I will speak to a little later in this chapter.

In addition to diet and exercise, the third contributor to my downward spiral of health was vitamin supplements. I am a strong advocate of alternative medicine and do believe that vitamin supplementation can be beneficial. In fact, my father included supplementation of Vitamin E in his regimen toward improved health. However, as with all things, be careful.

Any vitamin product has a chemical makeup, which reacts with your body's own chemistry, in a particular manner. The nature of this reaction is sometimes unknown due to insufficient scientific data obtained through controlled experiments.

One example of this for me was the use of soy. In general, protein is one of the basic substances our bodies need to thrive and grow. In particular soy protein has been touted as one of the most plentiful and healthful ways of meeting all of your body's protein needs. I have often times heard soy characterized in commercials advocating its use as miraculous – "the miracle of the soy bean". If you accept this premise, then vitamin supplements, which contain large quantities of soy, would certainly be thought of as a good thing.

The one thing that I was unaware of about soy was its potential affect on the thyroid gland. Some studies have shown that soy could have a detrimental affect on your thyroid gland. How could this wonder of nature, this "miracle" food, have a harmful effect on one of the body's key glands? The biochemistry behind the interaction between soy and the thyroid gland aren't clear to me, but the bottom line of potential harmful effects are.

I have been a strong believer in soy's benefits to the body. Coming from a family that had a history of heart disease, I was always looking for alternative sources of protein, other than red meat, since red meat is loaded with fat and cholesterol. Soy seemed to be just the ticket! At this point in my life, I was taking vitamin supplements as a regular course of action, in an effort to optimize my health. I took "E", "C", "B", amino acids, and many others, which were inclusive in a multi-vitamin, produced and distributed by a heart surgeon. It was at this time that I became aware of a vitamin supplement that had high levels of soy and "MSM" and was being touted as a new breakthrough in supplementation. Its claim to fame was that it would replenish the body of all its needed nutrients, robbed by the chemicals and the environment in our modern society. I was interested in giving this supplement a try. I thought, after all, Soy is a very "good" thing. I ceased taking the multi-vitamin and began taking these "soy" vitamins. My wife began taking them as well. After taking them for a few months we began to notice that we were feeling more sluggish and it even almost appeared that our teeth started turning green! We both immediately stopped taking them, and shortly after, our teeth resumed their normal bright white appearance, although our sluggishness did not go away.

This brings us to what I think was the fourth primary contributor to my spiral downward into disease. The colon has a tremendous affect on the overall health of the body. It removes the nutrients our body needs from digested food and transfers them to our body while removing any toxins and waste for proper disposal. If we consume contaminated food, we take the risk of harboring a parasite in this most pivotal element of our body's ecosystem. The effect of a parasite in the body can be quite detrimental. Unfortunately, it is rare to receive medical treatment for a parasitic invasion, because it is difficult to specifically determine if symptoms of the disease are directly attributed to a parasite.

The damage that a parasite can do to the body is quite devastating. It can throw off the entire immune system. The body will begin producing antibodies to attack this foreign invader. The only problem is that these guys are pretty clever and can disguise themselves to appear as normal body tissue. Hence, when the attack anti-bodies go after the invasive parasite with a search and destroy mission, normal body tissue becomes an innocent casualty. This in general is what an autoimmune disease is all about. The body's defense mechanism attacks itself and destroys perfectly good tissue. It is an unfortunate self-destructive cycle.

My wife and I had the blessing of being married at the Vatican in Italy and subsequently taking three weeks to honeymoon in Europe. However, after returning home, the both of us felt sluggish and had persistent bouts of diarrhea for approximately six months. This, we came to believe, was a direct result of picking up a parasite while we were in Europe. This feeling of sluggishness for such a long period was extremely out of character for the both of us. I mentioned that I was very active with running, biking and swimming. One of the things that attracted me to my wife so much was that she also was extremely active with both running and biking. Before we got married, we would hop on our bikes and ride fifty miles without even thinking twice about it. We were constantly on the go, with seemingly endless energy. Therefore, this sudden crash of our bodies, where we got tired just thinking about walking around the block let alone biking fifty miles, was extremely out of character.

When we travel abroad, we like to experience the character and flavor of each city we encounter. One large part of this experience is the food that each country or city has to offer. Whether it was eating a crepe' at a sidewalk stand along the Champs Elysees, or Bratwurst and Wiener Schnitzel in Salzburg, it is hard to say where we picked up our unfriendly parasite companion. In fact, it could have even been the fish, which was served on the plane on the flight home. It seemed that after eating that fish, the arrival and taxi to the terminal took an eternity. Once we made it to the terminal, the first and most urgent stop after getting through customs was the restroom. Something in that fish just did not agree with my body.

In summary, I attribute my spiral downward into disease to the four previously mentioned topics simply because they all coincidentally "climaxed" at approximately the same point in my life and they all "can" be direct contributors to the type of disease which I obtained.

In review, the potential four contributors to my disease were:

1) Low fat, high carbohydrate diet.

2) Excessive levels of exercise.

3) High intake of soy.

4) Parasites.

I will summarize how each of these can contribute to the onset of Hashimoto's Hypothyroidism.

Low Fat, high carbohydrate diet:

For a number of years before my Hashimoto's diagnosis, my diet was primarily low fat, high carbohydrate. My main staples were pasta and bread. I must have gotten this from my mother who is Italian. Of-course, coming from a Slovak heritage on my father's side, a favorite treat in my diet was also pierogi's. For those of you not familiar with peirogi's, they are kind of like big ravioli's with potato and cheese filling. Carbohydrates and foods with low fat, were just what the doctor ordered as far as I was concerned. Remember that my primary focus was reducing my fat and cholesterol intake for good cardiac health.

It has been only recently that I became aware of a thing called celiac disease. Celiac Disease is intolerance to gluten, where gluten is an element of wheat, rye, barley and oats. These were my main staples for years. I wonder if my excessive focus on these types of foods eventually built up an intolerance in my system. Most people who have celiac disease do not even know it, and it is rare that it is diagnosed.

Researchers and doctors alike have identified a specific link between celiac disease and hypothyroidism. Balch and Balch in Prescription for Nutritional Healing state, "Certain autoimmune disorders can also be associated with Celiac Disease,..., thyroid disease,.." Also a report in the medical journal, Digestive Disease and Sciences stated, "a significant number of patients with autoimmune thyroid disease also have celiac disease." What was most encouraging in this same report to sufferers of Hashimoto's Thyroiditis was the possibility of the disease being overcome. It stated, "...anti-gliadin antibodies and anti-endomysium antibodies disappear after 3 to 6 months of a gluten-free diet,...so do...organ specific autoantibodies." Believe me it's possible. My thyroid antibodies vamoosed from my body, as you will see a little later in this book. Whether the exodus of my antibodies was related to a change in my diet, or other factors that I will mention in subsequent chapters, is debatable. The bottom line is that they are gone!

In addition, I will address more specific details in the "Put Protein in your Diet" chapter relating to how a high carbohydrate, low protein diet, can work against promoting a strong Immune system. Contrary to what you might think, sufferers of Hashimoto's have a weakened immune system, not an immune system on steroids. Therefore, it appears that anything that can be done to strengthen the immune system, helps recovery from Hashimoto's.

High levels of exercise:

Intense levels of exercise, such as experienced with training for and participating in marathons, puts a strain on the body. This type of exertion has been shown to weaken the immune system making the body susceptible to immune system related disorders.

High Intake of Soy:

Intake of Soy has been shown to have a detrimental affect on the thyroid gland.

Soy has enlarged thyroids by decreasing iodine absorption from the intestine. In the 50's, babies allergic to milk who were fed soy formula, got goiters.

Since this phenomenon became known in the fifties, the medical profession's prevailing line of thought was that most American diets included a significant amount of iodine, thereby minimizing soy's affect in the onset of Hashimoto's. However, my personal experience is an argument against this line of thought, and continued research being done on the effect of soy has brought to light some startling conclusions.

The isflavones in soy are thought to be the primary anti-thyroid culprit. So much so, that researcher Dr. Mike Fitzpatrick is calling for the soy industry to remove isoflavones from their products. Another study done in the U.K. has shown that adults who consume soy products for an extended period of time run the risk of suppressing and enlarging the thyroid gland. In general, a word of caution is in order if you are a consumer of soy products, especially if you are also a sufferer of Hashimoto's.

Parasites:

I think that a parasite may have been the primary instigator in the onset of Hashimoto's in my body. Parasites can enter our body through contaminated food. Once they get into the intestinal tract, they can pass through the intestinal wall, into the blood stream. If you have poor digestion, undigested particles of food also pass into the blood stream, and serve as a food source for these annoying parasites. They will continue to grow, and kick off the body's defense mechanism (the immune system) to attack and destroy. The problem with these unwelcome invaders is that, once in the blood stream, they can disguise themselves as healthy body tissue, say for instance the thyroid gland. When the immune system sends out its antibodies to get rid of these buggers, it may take the thyroid gland along with them. The antibody's motto is to kill first, ask questions later. As a result, your thyroid is a casualty of your own attack against an invader.

DIAGNOSIS AND TREATMENT PLAN

Several months after my wife and I got back from our honeymoon, I went for my annual physical. All of my previous physicals had been fairly routine with never any cause for concern expressed by the physician. In fact, the norm was to receive praise and salutations for how good my health was. I attributed this to the previously mentioned regimen that I experienced from a young age, with diet and exercise.

However, this physical was to be different. After my visit, I received a letter in the mail from my doctor with a note and prescription. The note said that I was found to have an elevated level of TSH in my blood and that I should begin taking synthroid per the enclosed prescription. I was upset about the approach that this particular doctor took to inform me about a disease and his desire for me to begin taking a medication for every day of the rest of my life. If a Doctor is too busy to inform his patient about such a condition, then he/she is too busy and should perhaps re-evaluate his/her priorities. Nevertheless, the bombshell was dropped and I had to process this information.

First of all, I had no clue what TSH was, or for that matter what synthroid was. I could not understand why all of a sudden, I would have this thyroid disease, when I never had any previous indication of such a thing. I am not one to blindly accept things and just go along with things, like a cow being led to the slaughter. Since this doctor chose not to respect my intelligence and provide me the information I needed to make a decision about my health, I was forced to find the answers I needed on my own. Looking back, perhaps it was a Godsend to me that this doctor was disrespectful, because if he was respectful and presented a good case to me, I may have accepted his argument and been without any natural thyroid function today! Dependant on a chemical supplement for the rest of my life.

When I was told about the thyroid problem for the first time, my TSH level was 12.45. The blood work, which I had done for this physical, did not include a measure of thyroid anti-bodies. Those diagnosed with Hashimoto's are intimately aware of these annoying anti-bodies, as being the source of the disease. I have included a copy of this initial blood test report, carefully omitting any reference to any hospital and Physician. Reference figure (2).

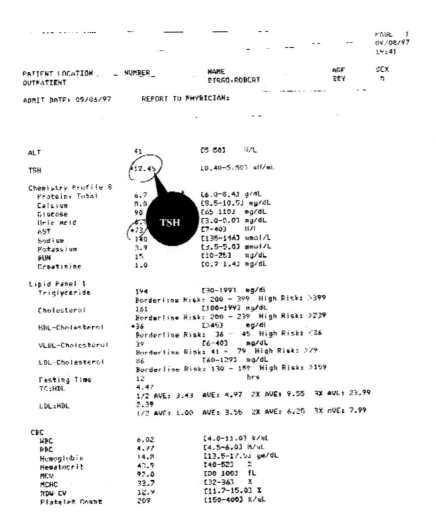

PATIENT LOCATION   _ NUMBER_   NAME   AGE   SEX
OUTPATIENT   DIRGO,ROBERT   38Y   M

ADMIT DATE: 09/06/97   REPORT TO PHYSICIAN:

ALT   41   [5-50]   U/L

TSH   12.45   [0.40-5.50] uU/mL

Chemistry Profile 8
  Protein, Total   6.7   [6.0-8.4] g/dL
  Calcium   8.9   [8.5-10.5] mg/dL
  Glucose   90   [65-110] mg/dL
  Uric Acid   6.7   [3.0-8.0] mg/dL
  AST   73   [7-40]   U/L
  Sodium   140   [135-146] mmol/L
  Potassium   3.9   [3.5-5.0] mmol/L
  BUN   15   [10-25]   mg/dL
  Creatinine   1.0   [0.7-1.4] mg/dL

Lipid Panel 1
  Triglyceride   194   [30-199] mg/dL
                        Borderline Risk: 200 - 399 High Risk: >399
  Cholesterol   161   [100-199] mg/dL
                        Borderline Risk: 200 - 239 High Risk: >239
  HDL-Cholesterol   36   [>45]   mg/dL
                        Borderline Risk: 36 - 45 High Risk: <36
  VLDL-Cholesterol   39   [6-40]   mg/dL
                        Borderline Risk: 41 - 79 High Risk: >79
  LDL-Cholesterol   86   [60-129] mg/dL
                        Borderline Risk: 130 - 159 High Risk: >159
  Fasting Time   12   hrs
  TC:HDL   4.47
                        1/2 AVE: 3.43 AVE: 4.97 2X AVE: 9.55 3X AVE: 23.99
  LDL:HDL   2.39
                        1/2 AVE: 1.00 AVE: 3.55 2X AVE: 6.26 3X AVE: 7.99

CBC
  WBC   6.02   [4.0-11.0] k/uL
  RBC   4.77   [4.5-6.0] M/uL
  Hemoglobin   14.8   [13.5-17.5] gm/dL
  Hematocrit   43.9   [40-52]   %
  MCV   92.0   [80-100] fL
  MCHC   33.7   [32-36]   %
  RDW-CV   12.9   [11.7-15.0] %
  Platelet Count   209   [150-400] k/uL

Figure 2

When I received this report, I was shocked, angry and depressed. Shocked because this was something that was totally unexpected. Angry because of how it was handled by the physician. Depressed because I was just married and could not believe that I was only now finding out about some health problems. What timing, I thought.

I began to do as much research as possible on the Thyroid gland, Hashimoto's Thyroiditis and synthroid. Having received a Bachelor's degree in Mechanical engineering, a Master's in Statistics, being three classes short of receiving a second Master's in Community Counseling and having a Phd in Operations Research halfway completed; I knew a little about doing Research. With the advent of the Internet, it is amazing how much information is now available to anyone with the time and patience to find it.

The one thing I came across in the research, which caused me concern about taking the synthroid, was from a University of Massachusetts study. It stated that, "...levthyroxine (Synthroid and others), can cause a loss of as much as 13 percent of bone mass." Now, I know as one gets older, the bones tend to weaken, so I had no interest whatsoever in trying to expedite the weakening process. If there was any other way to treat this problem, I wanted to find it.

I suppose my anger and disbelief of the doctor helped me rationalize not filling the synthroid prescription. Having a masters in Statistics, also helped me rationalize the test results. The inaccuracies, which are inherent in any test, could have given me a false positive! Did I want to start taking a drug for every day of the rest of my life that could have a negative impact on my bone mass as well as inactivate the production of the thyroid hormone from my thyroid gland, when I could have gotten a false positive? I don't think so!

I decided to work on changing my diet to improve my health and concurrently try to optimize my exercise regimen. (Although at this time I thought, optimize meant running another marathon.) After implementing these lifestyle changes, I decided that I would get another physical the following year to see how things had progressed. From a diet perspective,

I investigated a number of the current break-through diets, which were being promulgated on the market. One in particular, Protein Power, I will talk about further in a subsequent chapter.

In addition to diets, I began doing research into what foods were friendly to the Thyroid Gland. In Prescription for Nutritional Healing, Balch and Balch make the following recommendations, " molasses, egg yolks, parsley, apricots, dates, prunes, fish, chicken, raw milk and cheeses". I wondered if these were foods that I should strive to include in my diet, what foods should I avoid or include minimally. Again, referring to Balch and Balch: " brussel sprouts, peaches, pears, spinach, turnips, and cruciferous vegetables such as cabbage, broccoli, kale, and mustard greens". I have frequently tried to avoid processed foods in the past (i.e. potato chips, etc.) but I only accelerated my vigilance to avoid them after my diagnosis. My wife and I began drinking steam-distilled water in an effort to eliminate as many impurities as possible from our systems. Can you taste tap water and not wonder what is in it? Sometimes the chlorine is so strong, I wonder if the water line was misdirected through somebody's swimming pool.

Our family has tried to use organic or natural products as much as possible. One product that we have been using is Tom's toothpaste. One unique thing about this brand of toothpaste is that it does not have any fluoride. Why this is good news to Hashimoto's sufferers is that, "Chlorine and fluoride block iodine receptors in the thyroid gland, resulting in reduced iodine-containing hormone production and finally in hypothyroidism".

I began plotting my basal body temperature every morning. I checked my temperature under my armpit and plotted it on a chart. When I started the chart, most of my readings were below 97.6 F. However, I noticed improvement after several months of modifying my diet, and paying attention to factors that have a detrimental affect on the thyroid gland. I was able to get my basal body temperature above 97.6 F the majority of the time. I have included one of my charts (figure 3) which reflects the temperature progression.

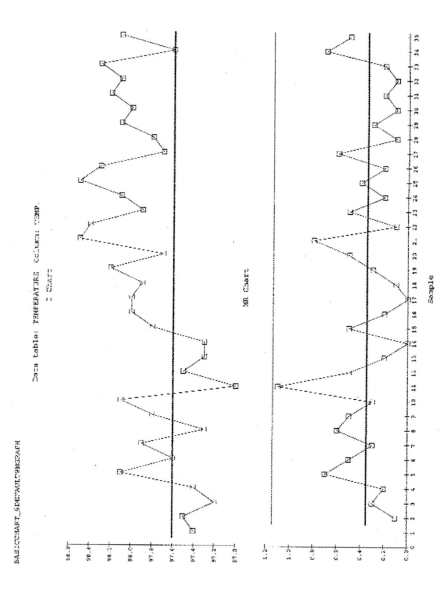

Figure 3

Having obtained some success with my basal temperature and feeling "better" physically after making some dietary and exercise changes, I thought that I must be on the right track. Surely, I thought, when I went for my next physical that the TSH level would be back to normal and this unfortunate diagnosis would be behind me.

As I mentioned before, I wanted to optimize my exercise regimen concurrently with improving my diet. However at this time in my life, I thought optimizing my exercise regimen meant running another marathon. So, I picked a marathon to run in the spring. This one was the Cleveland, Ohio marathon. I had a few months to train, which gave me plenty of time. I saw the training and the running of the marathon as being steps toward improving my thyroid condition. When one trains for a marathon, you have to log a lot of miles. Typically I would run the shorter distances during the week, whereby shorter, I mean three to six miles. On the weekends, I would put in the longer runs. The longer runs typically went from eight miles up to twenty-two miles. The marathon itself is twenty-six miles. I never have run the whole twenty-six miles when training for a marathon. So for several months I went through this regimen, week after week, until race day in Cleveland. I ran the race faster than I have done before and felt strong for most of the race. After finishing the race I felt elated. Surely this accomplishment could only support again that I was on the right track for overcoming my Thyroid problem. Besides, how could someone who truly has hypothyroidism be able to train for and complete a twenty-six mile grueling marathon road race?

My confidence level was high that I was doing something right. It was a year and a half now since my last physical, so I thought that I should schedule my next appointment for a physical. I just could not wait to see the results of the TSH level in my blood test. I imagined myself feeling somewhat smug about successfully overcoming this health issue.

The results came back. I have included the actual results of this second physical, in figure (4) and (5). This time the doctor not only ordered the TSH to be checked, but also requested that the thyroid antibodies be checked as well. It rather was like a good news-bad news thing when I got the results. The good news was that my TSH level dropped from the 12.45 of my last test to 10.59. I had mixed emotions. I thought certainly this was a step in the right direction, and if this disease is suppose to get progressively worse, how could my TSH level get lower without ever taking any synthroid? I hung on to this glimmer of hope, but I was still disappointed that the value was not closer to the high limit of the normal range.

The result that was the biggest shocker was the thyroid antibody measure. In my previous blood work this was not checked, so I had nothing to benchmark it against. However, it was way out! The normal range was 0 to 5 IU/ML and my result was 707! This was conclusive evidence to the doctor that I had Hashimoto's Thyroiditis. Otherwise known to us Hashi's as the autoimmune disease of the thyroid gland. He discounted the reduction of the TSH as not being significant, and because the antibody level was so high, he thought that I should immediately begin taking the synthroid.

LABORATORY REPORT

PATIENT LOCATION	NUMBER	NAME	AGE	SEX
		DIRGO, ROBERT	39Y	M

ADMIT DATE: 07/23/1999 REPORT TO PHYSICIAN:

Differential			
Neut%	57.8	[40-70]	%
Abs Neut	2.64	[1.8-7.7]	K/uL
Lymph%	29.5	[22-44]	%
Abs Lymph	1.35	[1.0-4.8]	K/uL
Mono%	*9.2	[0-7.0]	%
Abs Mono	0.42	[0-0.8]	K/uL
Eosin%	3.1	[0-4]	%
Abs Eosin	0.14	[0-0.4]	K/uL
Baso%	0.4	[0-1]	%
Abs Baso	0.07	[0-0.2]	K/uL
Fibrinogen	259	[200-400]	mg/dL
GGT	12	[0-50]	U/L
Lipid Panel 1			
Triglyceride	46	[30-199]	mg/dL
	Borderline Risk: 200 - 399 High Risk: >399		
Cholesterol	162	[100-199]	mg/dL
	Borderline Risk: 200 - 239 High Risk: >239		
HDL-Cholesterol	53	[>45]	mg/dL
	Borderline Risk: 36 - 45 High Risk: <36		
VLDL-Cholesterol	9	[6-40]	mg/dL
	Borderline Risk: 41 - 79 High Risk: >79		
LDL-Cholesterol	100	[60-129]	mg/dL
	Borderline Risk: 130 - 159 High Risk: >159		
Fasting Time	12		hrs
TC:HDL	3.06		
	1/2 AVE: 3.43 AVE: 4.97 2X AVE: 9.55 3X AVE: 23.97		
LDL:HDL	1.89		
	1/2 AVE: 1.00 AVE: 3.55 2X AVE: 6.25 3X AVE: 7.99		
APTT			
APTT	26.6	[21.5-32.5]	sec
T4/FTI			
T4	7.8	[5.0-11.0]	ug/dL
T4 Uptake	0.84	[0.70-1.20]	
FTI	9.3	[6.0-11.0]	ug/dL
TSH	*10.59	[0.40-5.50]	uU/mL

TSH

Figure 4

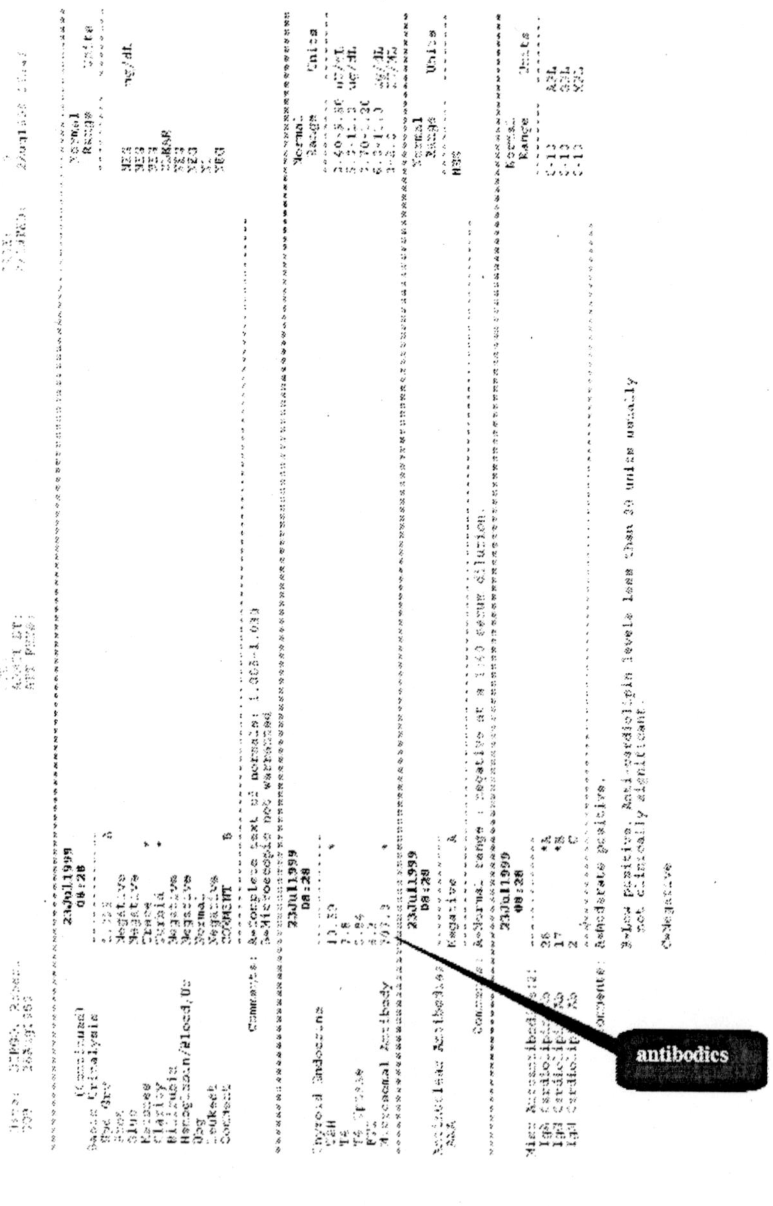

(Continued)	23Jul1999 08:28		Normal Range	Units
Basic Urinalysis				
Spc Grv	[illegible]	A		
Prot	Negative		NEG	mg/dL
Glu	Negative		NEG	
Ketones	Trace	*	NEG	
Clarity	Turbid	*	CLEAR	
Billirubin	Negative		NEG	
Hemoglobin/Blood,Ur	Negative		NEG	
Ubg	Normal		NL	
Leukest	Negative		NEG	
Comment	COMMENT	B		

Comments: A=Complete text of normals: 1.005-1.030
B=Microscopic not warranted

	23Jul1999 08:28		Normal Range	Units
Thyroid Endocrine				
TSH	10.30	*	0.40-5.50	uU/mL
T4	7.8		5.0-11.0	ug/dL
T4 Uptake	0.84		0.70-1.20	
FTI	6.2		6.0-11.0	ug/dL
Microsomal Antibody	707.3	*	0-2.0	IU/ML

	23Jul1999 08:28		Normal Range	Units
Antinuclear Antibodies				
ANA	Negative	A	NEG	

Comments: A=Normal range : negative at a 1:40 serum dilution.

	23Jul1999 08:28		Normal Range	Units
Misc Autoantibodies(2)				
IgA Cardiolipin Ab	26	*A	0-13	APL
IgG Cardiolipin Ab	17	*B	0-13	GPL
IgM Cardiolipin Ab	2	C	0-13	MPL

Comments: A=Moderate positive.

B=Low positive. Anti-cardiolipin levels less than 30 units usually not clinically significant.

C=Negative

Figure 5

I was stunned again, but this time closer to accepting that maybe I had a thyroid problem that I was going to have to treat with synthroid. I went so far this time as to fill my prescription for the synthroid, but I still was reluctant to take it. I remembered the studies on the bone mass loss and just did not like the idea of taking a drug for the rest of my life.

I began thinking this through a little further and it just did not make sense to me. Should I go ahead and take the drug when it does not make sense? The thing that bothered me the most was that synthroid does not correct the source of the problem with Hashimoto's (antibodies attacking the thyroid gland), it only addresses the symptom (high TSH). I work in the Aerospace Industry and make a living trying to identify root causes of problems in order to obtain an adequate corrective action. To me, the treatment to take the synthroid was a cop out and did absolutely nothing to identify the true root cause of the problem. What was causing my body's natural defense mechanisms to attack itself? Shouldn't that be determined and corrected? Wouldn't that be an appropriate corrective action? I am not interested in treating the symptom; I want to correct the problem.

I posed these questions to my doctor and did not receive a satisfying response. He basically said, that is just the way it is and there is no way of identifying the source of the antibody autoimmune attack. That seemed like a pretty lame response to me. It is the type of response I would not accept in my line of business. So, I most certainly was not going to accept it when it pertained to my health.

As a result, I decided again not to take the synthroid and set out on another journey of research and fact-finding to implement a more appropriate corrective action!

An Alternative Approach

I thought that there must be some Alternative Medicine solutions to Hashimoto's Thyroiditis. I began searching on the Internet and was blessed to find a site that pertained to all types of Thyroid issues, including Hashimoto's Thyroiditis. Within this site there was a reference for Doctor's who practice Alternative Medicine that might be effective for Thyroid disorders. I found a doctor that was close by and contacted him. He was an answer to prayer. I scheduled an appointment with him at the earliest available time slot. When my wife and I went to the Doctor's office, we were very impressed. At this time, he was working out of his combination office/home log cabin and it was out in the middle of nowhere. He had a huge organic garden next to his cabin and there were a bunch of kids running around. In essence, he impressed us as an old-time country doctor.

After explaining my condition and history to the Doctor, he gave me a couple of recommendations. He definitely advised against running marathons when trying to rejuvenate an already over-taxed immune system. The exertion that the marathon puts on the body and all of its systems would only work against any efforts to improve the immune system.

Secondly, he recommended against taking vitamin supplements. I happened to bring along the bottles of various vitamins I was taking at the time. It is somewhat funny now looking back, but my bag of vitamin bottles was a small grocery bag. It must have looked like I was taking a small pharmacy of vitamin supplements. His concern with taking vitamin supplements was that the foods you consume do not typically have just one vitamin in them. Rather these vitamins exist in the foods we eat along with a variety of other nutrients. So, your body needs the whole food in order to be properly nourished, and not a specific supplement. In addition, whether your body truly assimilates the "C" or zinc or whatever supplement you take properly is up for debate. Some may argue that the body does not assimilate the nutrients out of the supplement and that it justs passes through your system, adding no value to your health.

Thirdly, he recommended that I begin taking some nutrients that would promote my immune system and help assimilate the digestion process. In order to do this he recommended that I take Blue Green Algae, Digestive Enzymes, Acidophilus, Bifidus, co-enzyme Q-10 and garlic. In addition to starting this regimen he suggested that I cleanse my colon with one of the many colon cleanse solutions on the market. Now I never heard of Blue Green Algae before. The only Algae that I was aware of was the pond scum that collects on local ponds. I will speak about each of these things briefly.

Blue-Green Algae:

Blue Green Algae, otherwise known as *Aphanizomenon flos-aquae,* is an all natural living organism. It is one of the oldest living organisms. In fact, it is thought to have played a significant role in the creation and maintenance of the earth's ecosystem in the earlier years of creation. Algae is found in lakes, ponds and any stagnant body of water. All algae is not created equal. There is green algae, red algae and blue-green algae. Each has its unique characteristics. I am not familiar enough with the specifics of how they differ, so I will not address that here.

The algae that I am most familiar with is Blue-Green Algae. It is found in various places around the world. The primary hot spot for blue green algae is Upper Klamath Lake, in Oregon. This is literally the Mecca of Blue-Green algae. The reason Upper Klamath Lake is so special is the environment of the Lake. It is known as one of the most pristine lakes on the planet. Its beauty and ecological integrity is being preserved and protected by strict restrictions on the access and use of the Lake. It is this purity of the environment, which the algae grows in, that empowers this microscopic creature.

The makeup of the blue-green algae is thought to be nearly identical to that of a mother's breast milk. Breast milk is probably the closest thing to the perfect food. Designed to meet the nutritional needs of a newborn child, it consists of multiple vitamins and amino acids. It is very high in protein, one of the highest sources of protein in the food chain. One of Blue-Green Algae's most significant elements is its Chlorophyll content. It is my understanding that it is extremely high in Chlorophyll. Chlorophyll has been shown to have possible benefits in cancer prevention. In addition, the chlorophyll and all of the other characteristics of Blue-Green Algae appear to work in concert as a strong promoter of the body's immune system. This, of-course, is my primary motivator as a sufferer of Hashimoto's.

It appears to me that this algae contains a powerhouse of nutrients that may be beneficial to my body's systems. The system that interested me most was the immune system. To me, that was the "root cause" of my problem (Hashimoto's AutoImmune disorder), and I wanted to try anything that would help eliminate it.

In doing research on blue-green algae, I came across an interesting tid bit of information. I found out that there have been cases where intake of the algae has caused harmful health conditions. However, clearly this concern is only a real one if the algae you consume is high in neurotoxins. Therefore, since not all blue-green algae is equal, the consumer should exercise care in selecting an algae to include in his/her diet. Just make sure that the algae you choose is pure.

Digestive Enzymes:

Digestive Enzymes are one of the many different types of enzymes that exist. Every cell of the Human body contains enzymes. Digestive Enzymes help the body process food through the various stages of digestion. There are three primary types of digestive enzymes: protease, which breaks down protein, amylase, which breaks down starch, and lipase, which breaks down fat. Most foods have their naturally occurring enzymes compromised when they are cooked or stored for prolonged periods.

The potential problem that occurs when food gets into the intestinal tract without being properly digested is that these undigested food particles can get into the blood system, thereby prompting the body's immune system to attack and destroy these invaders. Those of us diagnosed with Hasimoto's do not want to unnecessarily burden our already overburdened immune system.

Therefore, if you are diagnosed with Hashimoto's it might make sense to take a Digestive Enzyme supplement to aid in the digestion process and prevent undigested particles from streaming into the blood stream.

Clearly, anything that helps process the food we eat through the intestinal tract will reduce the necessity of the immune system to attack undigested particles of food. This is an obvious plus to the person trying to build up their immune system.

Acidophilus and Bifidus:

Acidophilus also known as *Lactobacillus acidophilus* and Bifidus also known as *Lactobacillus bifidus* are what are referred to as friendly bacteria. You may be wondering how in the world could bacteria be friendly. These guys are given this reference because they do wonderful things for the upper and lower intestines. They are workhorses in defending the intestinal flora from intruders like organisms and destructive bacteria.

These friendly bacteria are sometimes inadvertently destroyed when we take an antibiotic to combat a cold or the flu. The problem is that the antibiotic aggressively destroys any presence of the cold or flu bacteria. But while doing so, it destroys the friendly bacteria along with it.

It is obvious that the benefit of these "friendly" bacteria is proper digestive functioning and the maintenance of a healthy intestinal flora. As mentioned before, digestive problems can lead to autoimmune disease. Therefore, the maintenance of a healthy intestinal flora may also contribute towards a healthy immune system. A desirable outcome for sufferers of Hashimoto's Hypothyroidism.

Coenzyme Q10:

Coenzyme Q10 is a vitamin type supplement that I became familiar with several years ago. It was being touted then as being a significant factor in the prevention of heart disease. With heart disease in my family, nothing goes by that can be beneficial without someone in our family finding out about it. Coenzyme Q10 is kind of like an antioxidant, which helps promote proper blood circulation. I remember reading years ago that Coenzyme Q10 taken in conjunction with vitamin "E" had been shown to significantly improve circulation and work towards prevention of cardiac disease. I found this interaction effect most interesting. Each of these supplements on there own are very good, but when they are tag teamed they pack a knockout punch.

I had a good feeling about coenzyme Q10 for several years, specifically for the reasons I previously stated. I only recently learned that I should appreciate it significantly more. The reason for this new found appreciation is the benefits that have been linked to the immune system and coenzyme Q10. It is my understanding that coenzyme Q10, especially when taken in conjunction with vitamin "E", had shown favorable results in the stimulation of the immune system.

Speaking from my own experience, there seems to be some benefit. I address a number of different things in this book that I personally did to boost my immune system. I am not certain which one of them or what combination benefited me. You be the judge.

Garlic:

To me, garlic is the most underrated food that exists. I remember growing up and my grandmother bringing over to our house strings full of cloves of garlic. She ate garlic regularly and so have my parents. I used to eat it more regularly and then I let it slip out of my diet. Nowadays it is so convenient to include garlic in my diet. There are a million different garlic supplements that appear to give you the benefit from the actual cloves without the odor problems.

Garlic is a great promoter of the immune system and excellent for blood flow.

As you can see, the things that my doctor recommended were all related to building up the immune system. That made sense to me. If your immune system is functioning improperly, then why not try to fix it!

At this point in dealing with this disease, I was willing to try anything. So, I implemented the Doc's suggestions. By that, I mean that I started taking Blue-Green Algae, Digestive Enzymes, Co-Enzyme Q-10, Acidolfulis, Bifidus and Garlic. I also continued taking vitamin E. I have been taking vitamin E for years and am a firm believer of its cardiac related health benefits. I also cut back the amount of exercise I was doing. Instead of training for a marathon, I only ran three to four miles three times a week. However, I also continued doing some weight training. The benefits of weight training will be expounded on slightly in the next chapter. My weight training consisted of lifting weights three times a week for one to one and one-half hour per session.

The Doc suggested that it takes about ninety days at a minimum to recognize a noticeable benefit. My understanding is that the body completely recycles the blood every ninety days. So, after about ninety to one hundred and twenty days, I scheduled another appointment to have my TSH and thyroid antibodies checked.

I was thrilled to find out the results. Reference figure (6) for the actual results. As you can see, my TSH dropped again, almost another 2 points to 8.83. However, the big news to me as a diagnosed sufferer of Hashimoto's Thyroiditis Hypothyroidism, was that my thyroid antibodies, which were 707 four months prior, were now nonexistent!

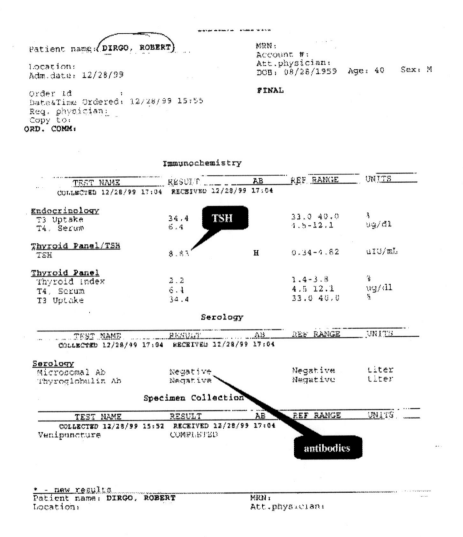

Figure 6

The root cause to my Hashimoto's, the autoimmune reaction of my body against the thyroid gland, has been overcome. And they said it couldn't be done! I was thankful to God for bringing this blessing into my life, and restoring my thyroid gland to proper functioning. It is no less than a miracle to me!

Therefore, in summary, I did the following things for several months to reverse my Hashimoto's Thyroiditis:

1) Follow the Protein Power plan.

2) Exercise regularly.
   Aerobic: (3) times/week
   Weight Training: (3) times/week

3) Colon Cleanse.

4) Supplement my diet with the following:
   Blue-Green Algae
   Digestive Enzymes
   Acidophilus
   Bifidus
   Coenzyme Q10
   Vitamin "E"
   Garlic

I cannot guarantee that you will have the same results as I did. My test results speak for themselves about my reversal of Hashimoto's. What I have outlined here is what I did between being diagnosed and obtaining my last blood test. I leave it to the reader to make his/her own judgements as to the value of what I did.

PUT PROTEIN IN YOUR DIET

I have been fortunate enough to be exposed to the work of Doctor Michael R. Eades and Doctor Mary Dan Eades through their published book, "Protein Power." What initially prompted me to buy their book was a desire to lose a spare tire I had around my waist. Which, by the way, I lost completely. I went from 205 lbs to 178 lbs. in about six to eight months. At 6'-2", 178 lbs., is just about my ideal weight. Not bad for someone suffering from Hashimoto's!

Protein Power burst onto the scene with mixed reviews. Their philosophy flew in the face of traditional thought. Could you imagine, a doctor suggesting that you can eat bacon, eggs and cheese to help lower your cholesterol, a mere ten years ago? I hardly think so. But that is exactly what these doctors ventured to preach with their Protein Power book.

Increasing the level of protein in my diet and reducing the number of carbohydrates, not only had the effect of ridding me of my spare tire, but also provided me with several other unexpected benefits.

Some of the claims of the Protein Power diet are that it creates an environment within your body that promotes increased circulation, greater oxygenation of your blood and a more balanced level of insulin. The optimization of eicasonoids and arachidonic acid are benefits I never even dreamed of. In fact, I never even heard of eicasonoids and arachidonic acid before reading this book. However, apparently their effect on the overall health and vitality of the body is vital. I will not detail the specifics of these benefits. You will have to read their book to find out.

I began on the Protein Power plan approximately six months before my second blood test. Recall in this test, there was a significant reduction in the TSH level (approximately 2 points). However, the thyroid antibodies were measured in this test and found to be extremely high. (707 vs. an acceptable range of 0 to 5)

I could argue that the benefits recognized in a reduction in TSH were directly or perhaps indirectly related to the Protein Power plan. Since I had no previous benchmark on the thyroid antibodies, I cannot really say that they got worse or better. I continued the Protein Power plan after the second blood test. At this time, I also incorporated Blue-Green Algae, Digestive Enzymes, Acidophilus, Bifidus and coenzyme Q10 into my diet. I continued with this entire regimen until the third blood test, which showed a significant reduction in TSH (approximately 2 points) as well as the elimination of thyroid antibodies. The elimination of Thyroid antibodies! I'm sorry, I felt like saying that again. It's music to the ears of someone diagnosed with Hashimoto's Thyroiditis Hypothyroidism.

So, for me it is hard to say if the Protein Power plan played a significant role or no role at all in the reversal of my disease. I think that it was all of the things I talk about in this book, interacting with one another, that gave me the benefits I experienced.

Whether it did or did not would have to be determined in a controlled scientific experiment. All I can say is that I am a believer in this approach to health.

HOLISTIC HEALTH

In the previous chapters, I have discussed primarily what I did to reclaim my health in regards to diet changes and diet supplements. I also mentioned in passing the affects of exercise on my condition. What I would like to do with this chapter is to pull it all together with other aspects of living that can significantly affect one's health. I believe that there are several essential aspects of living that should not be neglected if you want to maintain vibrant health. They are;

- ❖ Proper diet
- ❖ Drink lots of pure water
- ❖ Regular exercise
- ❖ Adequate Rest
- ❖ Stress Management

Proper Diet:

The proper diet, which worked for me in reversing my Hashimoto's, has been outlined in the previous chapters.

Drink Lots of Pure Water:

One of the essential things I did was to drink plenty of water. So much so that I felt like I was going to float. However, I did not drink just standard tap water. I have been drinking purified water, which has been through a reverse osmosis process, for quite some time now. I initially started with steam-distilled, but shortly changed to the reverse osmosis water. I thought it tasted better and accomplished the same objective as the distilled water.

The condition of tap water seems to be far from safe these days. It contains fluoride and chlorine, which both are thought to be unfriendly to the thyroid gland. In addition, numerous studies have shown that thousands of city water supplies across the country have been contaminated with various bacteria. So much so, that countless cases of illness have been directly associated with contaminated water supplies.

I am blessed to have a health-food store nearby where I get my supply of purified water from the reverse osmosis process. I am sure some day my wife and I will obtain our own reverse osmosis water purifier to meet our water needs.

Regular Exercise

I have spoken about the pros and cons of exercise throughout this book. One thing I feel that I have learned about exercise over the last few years is that weight training can play a significant role in my overall health. Coming from a family history of cardiac disease, I always felt that aerobic exercise was the optimum way to maintain vibrant health. In fact, I always thought weight training would work towards constricting blood vessels and indirectly promoting the onset of cardiac disease.

The recommendations by Eades and Eades in the Protein Power book and those made by Dr. Bob Arnot in "Dr. Bob Arnot's Guide to Turning Back the Clock," are very convincing of the overall benefits of weight training. My wife and I both have incorporated a weight-training regimen of one and one-half hours per day, three times per week into our overall exercise plan.

Running has been a favorite exercise for both my wife and me for quite a number of years. Its aerobic benefits are well documented and we both think it's fun! The key with running is balance. All things are good in moderation and running is no exception. Each persons balance point will be different. For my wife and I, we have incorporated three to four miles, three times a week into our exercise plan. My recommendation is to experiment to determine what works for you, and have FUN!

Adequate Rest:

Getting an adequate amount of rest is paramount for a healthy immune system. In fact, this is one factor that I failed to mention as a possible contributor to my spiral downward into disease. You see, I routinely got four hours, maybe five tops, of sleep each night. While obtaining this limited amount of rest, I pushed and worked my body and mind as much as possible. I have a love for life and strongly believe in living each and every minute to it's fullest potential.

However, this approach to living has its definite consequences. The primary one is a weakened immune system. Being diagnosed with Hashimoto's Thyroiditis Hypothyroidism was a wake up call for me. I changed my sleeping habits to help accentuate my efforts in recovering my health.

Most studies recommend that we should get eight hours of sleep each night for adequate health maintenance. Although, I made a commitment to increase the amount of sleep I get each night; I still have not gone that far. Now, I try to get seven hours of sleep a night. That seems to work good for me, and I firmly believe it has been a significant factor in my improved health.

Stress Management:

Last but most certainly not least is "Stress Management." Stress management will mean different things to different people. Everyone's stress level is different. Different things inflict stress on people. One person can experience stress if tasked with significant responsibility and another is stressed if not. Whatever your source of stress, you need to identify it and understand it. It is only then that you can begin to manage it.

Managing the stress in your life is just as unique as the stress itself is to each of us. To some, a quiet walk in the country or reading a book is a source of relief. To others, raging down a white-water river or para-sailing activities will be sources of relief. Again, it's paramount that you identify what works for you, and don't compromise yourself from indulging in that activity.

Above all, I think that it is critical that you foster a strong spirituality as the foundation of everything I have spoken about. To me, this is the greatest stress reducer. Our bodies are only temporal, but our spirits are everlasting. As important as it is to maintain the vibrant health of our bodies, our spirits are infinitely more important. In fact, I will go so far as to say that to truly obtain a healthy body is impossible without a healthy spirit. The two are inseparable. Mother Teresa spent hours each day in prayer. This was her source of energy. She once said, "in order to keep your light burning, you must keep filling it up."

In closing, I hope you have found this book useful in your battle to overcome your Hashimoto's disease. If not for a reversal of your disease, at least as an encouragement that there are possibilities that exist. Keep the faith, and never give up Hope!

PERSONAL HEALTH DIARY

Improving your health is not an easy thing to do, especially if you have Hashimoto's. However, it can be done. I found out that with the desire and will to seek out possible solutions, and implement them, I was able to turn my Hashimoto's around. I most certainly did not do it on my own without the proper direction of a physician. I just got a second opinion from a Doctor who was open-minded enough to consider alternative approaches to attack this disease. Everything I did was done under the direction of this physician.

One thing that you can do for yourself that may be beneficial is to keep a daily diary of the things you do to improve your health. This serves two purposes. One is to document your progress on your journey to improved health. When you look back at this journal after one week, then two and eventually three to four months, you will gain encouragement that you have stuck to your goal. The second is to establish a discipline for your health improvement efforts. More often than not, we find ourselves with our health predicaments because we have been undisciplined regarding our health. Make a plan and stick to it.

As an aide to help you establish this discipline, I have included in the following pages a Personal Health Diary. There were five main things that contributed to my recovery. They are **1) Diet (food & water), 2) Supplementation, 3) Exercise, 4) Adequate Rest and 5) Stress Management.** This diary is designed to record what you do for each of these categories on a daily basis. I've included enough diary sheets to cover three months of health improvement entries. Recall that I noticed some benefit in my case after four to six months. So you may have to make other arrangements for logging your status after the first three months, if necessary.

I wish you all the best in your efforts to improve your health. Remember that today is the first day of the rest of your life!

Personal Health Diary
Diet (food & water)
Week 1

Sunday_____

_____

_____

Monday_____

_____

_____

Tuesday_____

_____

_____

Wednesdayd_____

_____

_____

Thursday_____

_____

_____

Friday_____

_____

_____

Saturday_____

_____

_____

How I felt today:_____

_____

_____

_____

Personal Health Diary
Supplementation
Week 1

Sunday_____

_____

Monday_____

_____

Tuesday_____

_____

Wednesday_____

_____

Thursday_____

_____

Friday_____

_____

Saturday_____

_____

How I felt today:_____

_____

_____

_____

Personal Health Diary
Exercise
Week 1

Sunday_____

_____

_____

Monday_____

_____

_____

Tuesday_____

_____

_____

Wednesday_____

_____

_____

Thursday_____

_____

_____

Friday_____

_____

_____

Saturday_____

_____

_____

How I felt today:_____

_____

_____

_____

_____

Personal Health Diary
Adequate Rest
Week 1

Sunday_____
_____

Monday_____
_____

Tuesday_____
_____

Wednesday_____
_____

Thursday_____
_____

Friday_____
_____

Saturday_____
_____

How I felt today:_____
_____
_____
_____

Personal Health Diary
Stress Management
Week 1

Sunday_____

_____

_____

Monday_____

_____

_____

Tuesday_____

_____

_____

Wednesday_____

_____

_____

Thursday_____

_____

_____

Friday_____

_____

_____

Saturday_____

_____

_____

How I felt today:_____

_____

_____

_____

_____

Personal Health Diary
Diet (food & water)
Week 2

Sunday_____

_____

Monday_____

_____

Tuesday_____

_____

Wednesday_____

_____

Thursday_____

_____

Friday_____

_____

Saturday_____

_____

How I felt today:_____

_____

_____

_____

Personal Health Diary
Supplementation
Week 2

Sunday_____

_____

_____

Monday_____

_____

_____

Tuesday_____

_____

_____

Wednesday_____

_____

_____

Thursday_____

_____

_____

Friday_____

_____

_____

Saturday_____

_____

_____

How I felt today:_____

_____

_____

_____

_____

Personal Health Diary
Exercise
Week 2

Sunday_____

_____

Monday_____

_____

Tuesday_____

_____

Wednesday_____

_____

Thursday_____

_____

Friday_____

_____

Saturday_____

_____

How I felt today:_____

_____

_____

_____

Personal Health Diary
Adequate Rest
Week 2

Sunday_____

_____

_____

Monday_____

_____

_____

Tuesday_____

_____

_____

Wednesday_____

_____

_____

Thursday_____

_____

_____

Friday_____

_____

_____

Saturday_____

_____

_____

How I felt today:_____

_____

_____

_____

_____

Personal Health Diary
Stress Management
Week 2

Sunday_____

_____

Monday_____

_____

Tuesday_____

_____

Wednesday_____

_____

Thursday_____

_____

Friday_____

_____

Saturday_____

_____

How I felt today:_____

_____

_____

_____

Personal Health Diary
Diet (food & water)
Week 3

Sunday_____

_____

_____

Monday_____

_____

_____

Tuesday_____

_____

_____

Wednesday_____

_____

_____

Thursday_____

_____

_____

Friday_____

_____

_____

Saturday_____

_____

_____

How I felt today:_____

_____

_____

_____

_____

Personal Health Diary
Supplementation
Week 3

Sunday_____

_____

Monday_____

_____

Tuesday_____

_____

Wednesday_____

_____

Thursday_____

_____

Friday_____

_____

Saturday_____

_____

How I felt today:_____

_____

_____

_____

Personal Health Diary
Exercise
Week 3

Sunday_____

_____

_____

Monday_____

_____

_____

Tuesday_____

_____

_____

Wednesday_____

_____

_____

Thursday_____

_____

_____

Friday_____

_____

_____

Saturday_____

_____

_____

How I felt today:_____

_____

_____

_____

Personal Health Diary
Adequate Rest
Week 3

Sunday_____

_____

Monday_____

_____

Tuesday_____

_____

Wednesday_____

_____

Thursday_____

_____

Friday_____

_____

Saturday_____

_____

How I felt today:_____

_____

_____

_____

Personal Health Diary
Stress Management
Week 3

Sunday_____

_____

_____

Monday_____

_____

_____

Tuesday_____

_____

_____

Wednesday_____

_____

_____

Thursday_____

_____

_____

Friday_____

_____

_____

Saturday_____

_____

_____

How I felt today:_____

_____

_____

_____

_____

Personal Health Diary
Diet (food & water)
Week 4

Sunday_____

_____

Monday_____

_____

Tuesday_____

_____

Wednesday_____

_____

Thursday_____

_____

Friday_____

_____

Saturday_____

_____

How I felt today:_____

_____

_____

_____

Personal Health Diary
Supplementation
Week 4

Sunday_____

_____

_____

Monday_____

_____

_____

Tuesday_____

_____

_____

Wednesday_____

_____

_____

Thursday_____

_____

_____

Friday_____

_____

_____

Saturday_____

_____

_____

How I felt today:_____

_____

_____

_____

_____

Personal Health Diary
Exercise
Week 4

Sunday_____

_____

Monday_____

_____

Tuesday_____

_____

Wednesday_____

_____

Thursday_____

_____

Friday_____

_____

Saturday_____

_____

How I felt today:_____

_____

_____

_____

Personal Health Diary
Adequate Rest
Week 4

Sunday_____

_____

Monday_____

_____

Tuesday_____

_____

Wednesday_____

_____

Thursday_____

_____

Friday_____

_____

Saturday_____

_____

How I felt today:_____

_____

_____

_____

Personal Health Diary
Stress Management
Week 4

Sunday_____

_____

Monday_____

_____

Tuesday_____

_____

Wednesday_____

_____

Thursday_____

_____

Friday_____

_____

Saturday_____

_____

How I felt today:_____

_____

_____

_____

Personal Health Diary
Diet (food & water)
Week 5

Sunday_____

_____

_____

Monday_____

_____

_____

Tuesday_____

_____

_____

Wednesday_____

_____

_____

Thursday_____

_____

_____

Friday_____

_____

_____

Saturday_____

_____

_____

How I felt today:_____

_____

_____

_____

_____

Personal Health Diary
Supplementation
Week 5

Sunday_____

_____

Monday_____

_____

Tuesday_____

_____

Wednesday_____

_____

Thursday_____

_____

Friday_____

_____

Saturday_____

_____

How I felt today:_____

_____

_____

_____

Personal Health Diary
Exercise
Week 5

Sunday_____

_____

_____

Monday_____

_____

_____

Tuesday_____

_____

_____

Wednesday_____

_____

_____

Thursday_____

_____

_____

Friday_____

_____

_____

Saturday_____

_____

_____

How I felt today:_____

_____

_____

_____

_____

Personal Health Diary
Adequate Rest
Week 5

Sunday_____

_____

_____

Monday_____

_____

_____

Tuesday_____

_____

_____

Wednesday_____

_____

_____

Thursday_____

_____

_____

Friday_____

_____

_____

Saturday_____

_____

_____

How I felt today:_____

_____

_____

_____

_____

Personal Health Diary
Stress Management
Week 5

Sunday_____

_____

_____

Monday_____

_____

_____

Tuesday_____

_____

_____

Wednesday_____

_____

_____

Thursday_____

_____

_____

Friday_____

_____

_____

Saturday_____

_____

_____

How I felt today:_____

_____

_____

_____

_____

Personal Health Diary
Diet (food & water)
Week 6

Sunday_____

_____

_____

Monday_____

_____

_____

Tuesday_____

_____

_____

Wednesday_____

_____

_____

Thursday_____

_____

_____

Friday_____

_____

_____

Saturday_____

_____

_____

How I felt today:_____

_____

_____

_____

Personal Health Diary
Supplementation
Week 6

Sunday_____

_____

_____

Monday_____

_____

_____

Tuesday_____

_____

_____

Wednesday_____

_____

_____

Thursday_____

_____

_____

Friday_____

_____

_____

Saturday_____

_____

_____

How I felt today:_____

_____

_____

_____

Personal Health Diary
Exercise
Week 6

Sunday_____

_____

Monday_____

_____

Tuesday_____

_____

Wednesday_____

_____

Thursday_____

_____

Friday_____

_____

Saturday_____

_____

How I felt today:_____

_____

_____

_____

Personal Health Diary
Adequate Rest
Week 6

Sunday_____

_____

_____

Monday_____

_____

_____

Tuesday_____

_____

_____

Wednesday_____

_____

_____

Thursday_____

_____

_____

Friday_____

_____

_____

Saturday_____

_____

_____

How I felt today:_____

_____

_____

_____

_____

Personal Health Diary
Stress Management
Week 6

Sunday_____

_____

_____

Monday_____

_____

_____

Tuesday_____

_____

_____

Wednesday_____

_____

_____

Thursday_____

_____

_____

Friday_____

_____

_____

Saturday_____

_____

_____

How I felt today:_____

_____

_____

_____

_____

Personal Health Diary
Diet (food & water)
Week 7

Sunday_____

_____

_____

Monday_____

_____

_____

Tuesday_____

_____

_____

Wednesday_____

_____

_____

Thursday_____

_____

_____

Friday_____

_____

_____

Saturday_____

_____

_____

How I felt today:_____

_____

_____

_____

Personal Health Diary
Supplementation
Week 7

Sunday_____

_____

_____

Monday_____

_____

_____

Tuesday_____

_____

_____

Wednesday_____

_____

_____

Thursday_____

_____

_____

Friday_____

_____

_____

Saturday_____

_____

_____

How I felt today:_____

_____

_____

_____

_____

Personal Health Diary
Exercise
Week 7

Sunday_____

_____

Monday_____

_____

Tuesday_____

_____

Wednesday_____

_____

Thursday_____

_____

Friday_____

_____

Saturday_____

_____

How I felt today:_____

_____

_____

_____

Personal Health Diary
Adequate Rest
Week 7

Sunday_____

_____

Monday_____

_____

Tuesday_____

_____

Wednesday_____

_____

Thursday_____

_____

Friday_____

_____

Saturday_____

_____

How I felt today:_____

_____

_____

_____

Personal Health Diary
Stress Management
Week 7

Sunday_____

_____

_____

Monday_____

_____

_____

Tuesday_____

_____

_____

Wednesday_____

_____

_____

Thursday_____

_____

_____

Friday_____

_____

_____

Saturday_____

_____

_____

How I felt today:_____

_____

_____

_____

Personal Health Diary
Diet (food & water)
Week 8

Sunday_____

_____

_____

Monday_____

_____

_____

Tuesday_____

_____

Wednesday_____

_____

Thursday_____

_____

Friday_____

_____

_____

Saturday_____

_____

_____

How I felt today:_____

_____

_____

_____

Personal Health Diary
Supplementation
Week 8

Sunday_____

_____

_____

Monday_____

_____

_____

Tuesday_____

_____

_____

Wednesday_____

_____

_____

Thursday_____

_____

_____

Friday_____

_____

_____

Saturday_____

_____

_____

How I felt today:_____

_____

_____

_____

Personal Health Diary
Exercise
Week 8

Sunday_____

_____

Monday_____

_____

Tuesday_____

_____

Wednesday_____

_____

Thursday_____

_____

Friday_____

_____

Saturday_____

_____

How I felt today:_____

_____

_____

_____

Personal Health Diary
Adequate Rest
Week 8

Sunday_____

_____

Monday_____

_____

Tuesday_____

_____

Wednesday_____

_____

Thursday_____

_____

Friday_____

_____

Saturday_____

_____

How I felt today:_____

_____

_____

_____

Personal Health Diary
Stress Management
Week 8

Sunday_____

_____

_____

Monday_____

_____

_____

Tuesday_____

_____

_____

Wednesday_____

_____

_____

Thursday_____

_____

_____

Friday_____

_____

_____

Saturday_____

_____

_____

How I felt today:_____

_____

_____

_____

_____

Personal Health Diary
Diet (food & water)
Week 9

Sunday_____

_____

_____

Monday_____

_____

_____

Tuesday_____

_____

_____

Wednesday_____

_____

_____

Thursday_____

_____

_____

Friday_____

_____

_____

Saturday_____

_____

_____

How I felt today:_____

_____

_____

_____

Personal Health Diary
Supplementation
Week 9

Sunday_____

_____

Monday_____

_____

Tuesday_____

_____

Wednesday_____

_____

Thursday_____

_____

Friday_____

_____

Saturday_____

_____

How I felt today:_____

_____

_____

_____

Personal Health Diary
Exercise
Week 9

Sunday_____

_____

_____

Monday_____

_____

_____

Tuesday_____

_____

_____

Wednesday_____

_____

_____

Thursday_____

_____

_____

Friday_____

_____

_____

Saturday_____

_____

_____

How I felt today:_____

_____

_____

_____

Personal Health Diary
Adequate Rest
Week 9

Sunday_____

_____

_____

Monday_____

_____

_____

Tuesday_____

_____

_____

Wednesday_____

_____

_____

Thursday_____

_____

_____

Friday_____

_____

_____

Saturday_____

_____

_____

How I felt today:_____

_____

_____

_____

_____

Personal Health Diary
Stress Management
Week 9

Sunday_____

_____

_____

Monday_____

_____

_____

Tuesday_____

_____

_____

Wednesday_____

_____

_____

Thursday_____

_____

_____

Friday_____

_____

_____

Saturday_____

_____

_____

How I felt today:_____

_____

_____

_____

_____

Personal Health Diary
Diet (food & water)
Week 10

Sunday_____

_____

Monday_____

_____

Tuesday_____

_____

Wednesday_____

_____

Thursday_____

_____

Friday_____

_____

Saturday_____

_____

How I felt today:_____

_____

_____

_____

Personal Health Diary
Supplementation
Week 10

Sunday_____

_____

Monday_____

_____

Tuesday_____

_____

Wednesday_____

_____

Thursday_____

_____

Friday_____

_____

Saturday_____

_____

How I felt today:_____

_____

_____

_____

Personal Health Diary
Exercise
Week 10

Sunday_____

_____

_____

Monday_____

_____

_____

Tuesday_____

_____

_____

Wednesday_____

_____

_____

Thursday_____

_____

_____

Friday_____

_____

_____

Saturday_____

_____

_____

How I felt today:_____

_____

_____

_____

_____

Personal Health Diary
Adequate Rest
Week 10

Sunday_____

_____

_____

Monday_____

_____

_____

Tuesday_____

_____

_____

Wednesday_____

_____

_____

Thursday_____

_____

_____

Friday_____

_____

_____

Saturday_____

_____

_____

How I felt today:_____

_____

_____

_____

Personal Health Diary
Stress Management
Week 10

Sunday_____

_____

Monday_____

_____

Tuesday_____

_____

Wednesday_____

_____

Thursday_____

_____

Friday_____

_____

Saturday_____

_____

How I felt today:_____

_____

_____

_____

_____

Personal Health Diary
Diet (food & water)
Week 11

Sunday_____

_____

Monday_____

_____

Tuesday_____

_____

Wednesday_____

_____

Thursday_____

_____

Friday_____

_____

Saturday_____

_____

How I felt today:_____

_____

_____

_____

Personal Health Diary
Supplementation
Week 11

Sunday_____

_____

Monday_____

_____

Tuesday_____

_____

Wednesday_____

_____

Thursday_____

_____

Friday_____

_____

Saturday_____

_____

How I felt today:_____

_____

_____

_____

Personal Health Diary
Exercise
Week 11

Sunday_____

_____

_____

Monday_____

_____

_____

Tuesday_____

_____

_____

Wednesday_____

_____

_____

Thursday_____

_____

_____

Friday_____

_____

_____

Saturday_____

_____

_____

How I felt today:_____

_____

_____

_____

_____

Personal Health Diary
Adequate Rest
Week 11

Sunday_____

_____

Monday_____

_____

Tuesday_____

_____

Wednesday_____

_____

Thursday_____

_____

Friday_____

_____

Saturday_____

_____

How I felt today:_____

_____

_____

_____

Personal Health Diary
Stress Management
Week 11

Sunday_____

_____

_____

Monday_____

_____

_____

Tuesday_____

_____

_____

Wednesday_____

_____

_____

Thursday_____

_____

_____

Friday_____

_____

_____

Saturday_____

_____

_____

How I felt today:_____

_____

_____

_____

Personal Health Diary
Diet (food & water)
Week 12

Sunday_____

_____

Monday_____

_____

Tuesday_____

_____

Wednesday_____

_____

Thursday_____

_____

Friday_____

_____

Saturday_____

_____

How I felt today:_____

_____

_____

_____

_____

Personal Health Diary
Supplementation
Week 12

Sunday_____

_____

_____

Monday_____

_____

_____

Tuesday_____

_____

_____

Wednesday_____

_____

_____

Thursday_____

_____

_____

Friday_____

_____

_____

Saturday_____

_____

_____

How I felt today:_____

_____

_____

_____

_____

Personal Health Diary
Exercise
Week 12

Sunday_____
_____

Monday_____
_____

Tuesday_____
_____

Wednesday_____
_____

Thursday_____
_____

Friday_____
_____

Saturday_____
_____

How I felt today:_____
_____
_____
_____

Personal Health Diary
Adequate Rest
Week 12

Sunday_____

_____

_____

Monday_____

_____

_____

Tuesday_____

_____

_____

Wednesday_____

_____

_____

Thursday_____

_____

_____

Friday_____

_____

_____

Saturday_____

_____

_____

How I felt today:_____

_____

_____

_____

Personal Health Diary
Stress Management
Week 12

Sunday_____

_____

_____

Monday_____

_____

_____

Tuesday_____

_____

_____

Wednesday_____

_____

_____

Thursday_____

_____

_____

Friday_____

_____

_____

Saturday_____

_____

_____

How I felt today:_____

_____

_____

_____

CONCLUSIONS

I have since had one more blood test to evaluate my Thyroid condition. This latest one occurred approximately eight months after my previous test. I was pleased to see that my TSH continued to drop. The latest reading was 7.48. It dropped about another 1 and one-half points. There still was no evidence of any antibodies and I was also happy to find out that all traces of a goiter were gone. This latest test gives me encouragement that I must be doing something right for myself.

Over the past three years since implementing my Alternative approach to dealing with Hashimoto's, my TSH level has dropped about five points, my level of antibodies dropped from 707 to being non-existent and my goiter has vanished. Some may argue that obtaining a TSH level of 7.48 is not something to get excited about. The reason for this is that some experts' think that a TSH level above 5.5 is definitely Hypothyroidism. However, part of the controversy with TSH levels these days is assigning an appropriate outcome to the measure. Namely, what TSH number correlates to Hypothyroidism? Is hypothyroidism black and white, such that you have the disease if your TSH value is one one-hundredth of a point higher then a magic number? Or does one one-hundredth of a point lower indicate that you don't? If not one one-hundredth of a point then is it one-tenth or one whole point? Maybe it's two points or three! It seems to me that there are as many expert opinions on this matter as there are possibilities. Some believe that Hypothyroidism is not truly set in until the TSH is above 10.0. Others have said that a TSH above 2.0 in women is sufficient enough to negatively affect a women's fertility.

I had one doctor who thought my TSH of 10.45 accompanied by an antibody level of 707 definitely required treatment with the synthetic hormone, synthroid. Another thought that I was not even close to the point where I would want to start synthroid.

The bottom line to me is my personal health and quality of life. I live a very fulfilling life. I work as a Quality Manager in an Aerospace company, am Founder and President of an all-volunteer non-profit corporation, which has approximately 350 volunteers, am married to a beautiful and talented wife who is the love of my life. We run about three miles, three times a week, weight train and live a very active life. I'm not depressed, overweight, cold all the time, or lacking energy. Does my TSH mean I have Hypothyroidism? Maybe so, maybe no. If the experts can't seem to agree on this point, who am I to make a declarative statement.

In general it seems the majority of health professionals hold the opinion that a TSH above 5.5 indicates Hypothyroidism and it should be treated with some type of artificial hormone. In my case, the described symptoms of Hypothyroidism are not affecting my lifestyle. I by nature am reluctant to take any medication, especially if I can't recognize any of the symptoms the medication is supposed to fix.

If I had symptoms that were debilitating my lifestyle and my only option to fix them was to take a thyroid hormone supplement, natural or synthetic, then I would not hesitate to do so. I haven't reached that point yet. I suppose my TSH numbers seem to belie what I am saying, but to me that takes us back to the TSH controversy. What does this number mean?

The bottom line is that your health is your responsibility. You need to become as knowledgeable as possible about your disease, and find the best doctor for your personal situation. For you that may mean a treatment of synthetic or natural hormone replacement, or perhaps some alternative method. Whatever it is do not settle for less than regaining your health back and living life to the fullest.

When I go for my next blood test I believe that I will continue to see improvement in my TSH level and the antibodies will still be nonexistent.

However, if that is not the case, and my TSH is higher along with a recurrence of antibodies, then I will have to re-evaluate my situation. I will continue to pursue alternative methods of treatment until I think my options are limited to taking a thyroid supplement. Please feel free to contact me to find out if my successful treatment of Hashimoto's continues.

ABOUT THE AUTHOR

The Author resides in a suburb of Cleveland, Ohio with his charming wife Mary. He was listed in the International Who's Who of Professionals in 1997. He has spent most of his professional life in the Aerospace Industry, working in the realm of Quality Assurance. He has a Bachelors of Science degree in Mechanical Engineering and a Masters' degree in Statistics. He also has completed additional graduate course work; nearly completing a second master's degree in Community Counseling and half of the course work required for a Phd. in Operations Research. He has received the recognition of being certified by the American Society of Quality as a Certified Quality Engineer and a Certified Quality Auditor.

In addition to these accomplishments, he is also the President and Founder of the all-volunteer non-profit corporation, Gennesaret, Inc. Gennesaret is headquartered in Akron, Ohio. Its primary purpose is to provide transitional housing to two-parent families and supportive services to the poor.

For his efforts with this non-profit corporation he received the JC Penney Golden Rule Award in 1994, was nominated for the President of the United States Service Award in 1995, received an award for being the 1996 Ohio Outstanding Volunteer Administrator for Public or Private Non-Profit Organizations and was nominated for the National Ernst & Young, Entrepreneur of the Year Award in 1996.

If you would like to contact the author for further information, you can do so at *http://www.thyroid.bizland.com* or through the non-profit corporation. Its web address is *http:\\www.gennesaret.cc* Just click on the e-mail icon and mention that your inquiry is to Bob Dirgo in the body of the text. You can leave a phone message at 330-253-0011. Or write to;

Gennesaret, Inc.
Attn: Bob Dirgo
P.O. Box 4933
Akron, Ohio 44310

RESOURCES

In order to equip yourself with strategies and an understanding of the disease it is important to learn as much as possible. I was pleased to find out just how much information existed on Thyroid Disease an Hashimoto's in particular. There are a number of organizations that focus on Thyroid oriented issues. Contacting them can be quite helpful in answering some questions. However there are resources of all types out there; books, medical journals, internet web sites, videos, etc.

What I wanted to do was to provide you with a head start in gathering this information. I've compiled a list of resources that address the Thyroid and have shared it with you in the following pages. This type of information is subject to change, so please don't get frustrated if you find that a phone number or address has changed. I hope you find this beneficial.

Thyroid Related Organizations

Thyroid Foundation of America
Ruth Sleeper Hall RSL 350
40 Parkman Street
Boston, MA 02114-2698
Phone: 617-726-8500; 800-832-8321
Fax: 617-726-4136

National Graves' Disease Foundation
2 Tsitsi Court
Brevard, NC 28712
Phone: 704-877-5251
Fax: 704-877-5251

The Thyroid Society
7515 South Main Street, Suite 545
Houston, TX 77030
Phone: 713-799-9909

CHAPS (Congenital Hypothyroidism And Parent Support)
A Division of the Magic Foundation
1327 North Harlem Avenue
Oak Park, IL 60302
800-3-Magic-3
800-362-4423

Addison News
6142 Territorial Road
Pleasant Lake, MI 49272

American Autoimmune Related Diseases Assoc., Inc.
Michigan National Bank bldg.
15475 Gratiot Ave.
Detroit, MI 48205
Phone: 313-371-8600
Fax: 313-371-6002

International Council for Control of Iodine Deficiency Disorders
Box 511, University of Virginia Medical Center
Charlottesville, VA 22908

Magic Foundation
1327 North Harlem Avenue
Oak Park, IL 60302
Phone: 800-3-Magic-3

American Foundation for Thyroid Patients
P.O. Box 820195
Houston, TX 77282

Thyroid Society for Education and Research
7515 South Main Street, Suite 545
Houston, TX 77030
Phone: 1-800-Thyroid
Fax: 713-799-9919

Thyroid Cancer Survivor's Organization and Conference
P.O. Box 1545
New York, NY 10159-1545
Phone: 877-588-7904
Fax: 503-905-9725

International Organizations

Thyroid Foundation of Canada
96 Mack Street
Kingston, Ontario K7L 1N9 Canada
Phone: 613-544-8364
Fax: 613-544-9731

The British Thyroid Foundation
P.O. Box 97
Clifford Wetherby
West Yorks LS23 6XD United Kingdom

Thyroid Eye Disease Association
34 Fore Street
Chudleigh Devon
TQ13 OHX United Kingdom
Phone: 44-1626-852980
Fax: 44-1626-852980

Forum Schilddrtise e. V.
Anna-Birle-Strasse 1 (AM Petersweg)
D-55252 Wiesbaden/Mainz-Kastel
Germany

Schildklierstichting Nederland
Postbus 138
1620 AC Hoom
Nederlands

Thyroid Australia
PO Box 2575
Fitzroy Delivery Centre Melbourne
VIC 3065, Australia
Phone: 61-3-9561-3483
Fax:61-3-9561-7073

Australian Thyroid Foundation
P.O. Box 186
Westmead NSW 2145 Australia

Phone: 02-9890-6962
Fax: 02-9755-7073

Latin American Thyroid Society
Endocrinology/Medicine
Escola Paulista de Medicina
Universidade Federal de Sao Paulo
Caixa Postal 20266
04034-970 Sao Paulo, SP, Brazil
Phone: 55-11-571-9826
Fax: 55-11-575-0311

Physician Orientated Organizations

American Thyroid Association, Inc.
Montefiore Medical Center
111 East 210th Street
Bronx, NY 10467
Phone: 718-882-6047
Fax: 718-882-6085

American Association of Clinical Endocrinologists
701 Fisk St.
Suite 100
Jacksonville, FL 32204
Phone: 904-353-7878
Fax: 904-353-8185

The Endocrine Society
4350 East West Highway
Suite 500

Bethesda, MD 20814-4410
Phone: 301-941-0200
Fax: 301-941-0259

Endocrine Nurse's Society
P.O. Box 229
West Linn, OR 97068
Phone: 503-494-3714

American Society of Cytopathology
400 West 9th Street, Suite 201
Wilmington, DE 19801
Phone: 302-429-8802
Fax: 302-429-8807

Asia and Oceanic Thyroid Association
Department of Nuclear Medicine
Kyoto University of School of Medicine
Kyoto 606-01, Japan
Phone: 81-958-49-7260
Fax: 81-958-49-7270

The following is a listing of books that may be helpful in learning about the Thyroid and how it is affected.

Suggested Reading

Your Thyroid.
Lawrence C. Wood, et al, / Published 1995

The Thyroid Sourcebook: Everything You need to Know
M. Sara Rosenthal, Robert Volpe / Published 1996.

Could it be my Thyroid.
Sheldon Rubenfeld, et al / Published 1996

Hypothyroidism: The Unsuspected Illness.
Broda Otto Barnes, Broda O. Barnes / Published 1982

Prescription for Nutritional Healing.
James F. Balch and Phyllis A. Balch / Published 1997

Living Well with Hypothyroidism.
Mary J. Shomon / Published 2000

Sticking Out Our Necks.
Mary J. Shomon / Published 1999

How Your Thyroid Works.
H. Jack Baskin / Published 1991

Thyroid Disease, The Facts.
R.I. Bayliss, M.D. / Published 1982

The Thyroid Gland: A Book for Thyroid Patirnts.
Dr. Hamburger. / Published 1991

The Thyroid Sourcebook.
M. Sara Rosenthal.

The Thyroid Book: What Goes Wrong and How to Treat It.
    Martin I. Surks / Published 1994

The Thyroid Book
    Martin I. Surks, M.D.

The Thyroid Solution: A Mind-Body Program for Beating Depression and Regaining Your Emotional and Physical Health.
    Ridha Arem, M.D.

Solved: The Riddle of Illness.
    Stephen Langer, M.D. and James F. Scheer.

Protein Power.
    Eades and Eades. / Published 1995.

Turning Back the Clock.
    Dr. Bob Arnot / Published 1994

The Thyroid Gland. (Video)
    Dr. C. Everett Koop

The Immune System Cure
    Vanderhaeghe & Bolic / 1999

The following is a list of Internet sites which relate to Thyroid disease.

Internet Sites.

1) *http://www.thyroid-info.com*

2) *http://home.ican.net/~thyroid/English/Guides.html*

3) *http://www.thyroid.com/index.html*

4) *http://www.thyroid.org/*

5) *http://www.healthy.net/asp/templates/article.asp?PageType= Article&ID=528*

6) *http://thyroidfoundation.org/*

7) *http://www.familyvillage.wisc.edu/lib_thyr.htm*

8) *http://www.my4tune.u-net.com/index.html*

9) *http://www.sarahealth.com/*

10) *http://www.methodisthealth.com/endocrin/tests.htm*

11) *http://www.ncl.ac.uk/child-health/guides/clinks2t.htm#thyroid*

12) *http://www.members.tripod.com/~TDmagicmom/index.html*

13) *http://www.users.fast.net/~sttaylor/*

14) *http://www.thyrolink.com/data/welcome.htm*

15) *http://www.tsh.org/*

16) *http://home.ican.net/~thyroid/Canada.html*

17) *http://www.thyroid-fed.org/*

REFERENCES

Chapter 1:
Endocrine Disorders & Endocrine Surgery
    http://www.endocrineweb.com
Koop, C. Everett, et.al. "Thyroid Disorders: at time of diagnosis."
    Time Life Medical, 1996.
Santa Monica Thyroid Diagnostic Center
    http://www.thyroid.com/fun-stuff.html
Thyroid Home Page
    http://www.thyroid.com/patient.html
Thyroid Gland Disease, Conditions and all treatment options
    http://www.thyroid.net
Wood, Lawrence and David Cooper and E. Chester Ridgway.
    Your Thyroid. NY: Ballantine, 1995.

Chapter 2:
Balch, James and Phyllis Balch. *Prescription for Nutritional Healing.*
    NY: Avery, 1997.
Berti, Irene et al. "Usefulness of Screening Program for Celiac
    Disease in Autoimmune Thyroiditis." Digestive Diseases
    and Sciences, February 2000; 45: 403-406.
Shomon, Mary J., *Living Well with Hypothyroidism.*
    N.Y.: Avon, 2000.
Thyroid Disease.
    http://thyroid.about.com/health/thyroid/library/
    weekly/aa083099.htm

Wood, Lawrence and David Cooper and E. Chester Ridgway.
    Your Thyroid. NY: Ballantine, 1995.

Chapter 3:
    Balch, James and Phyllis Balch. *Prescription for Nutritional Healing.*
    NY: Avery, 1997.

Chapter 4:
    Balch, James and Phyllis Balch. *Prescription for Nutritional Healing.*
    NY: Avery, 1997.
    Goering, Laurie. "Death by pond scum: blue-green neurotoxin".
    The Seattle Times 7 December 1997.

Chapter 5:
    Eades, Michael and Mary Dan Eades. *Protein Power.*
    NY: Bantam, 1996.

Chapter 6:
    Arnot, Bob. *Dr. Bob Arnot's Guide to Turning Back the Clock.*
    Canada: Little, Brown & Company, 1995
    Eades, Michael and Mary Dan Eades. *Protein Power.*
    NY: Bantam, 1996.
    Vanderhaeghe & Bouic, *The Immune System Cure.*
    N.Y.: Kensington, 1999.